Mental Strategies to Defeat Diet Hunger and Junk Food Cravings

Lose Weight and Keep It Off By Transforming the Mind & Behaviors Volume 2

ROBERT DAVE JOHNSTON

Published by:

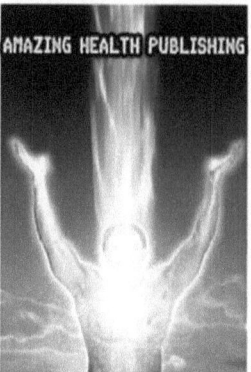

If you are interested in reading the next volume, follow Rob on Twitter @FitnessFasting

Copyright

Disclaimer & Legal Notices

The health-related information and suggestions contained in any of the books or written material mentioned above are based on the research, experience and opinions of the Author and other contributors. Nothing herein should be misinterpreted as actual medical advice, such as one would obtain from a Physician, or as advice for self-diagnosis or as any manner of prescription for self-treatment.

Neither is any information herein to be considered a particular or general cure for any ailment, disease or other health issue. The material contained within is offered strictly and solely for the purpose of providing Holistic health education to the general public. Persons with any health condition should consult a medical professional before entering this or any fasting, weight loss, detoxification or health related program.

Even if you suffer from no known illness, we recommend that you seek medical advice before starting any fasting, weight loss and/or detoxification program, and before choosing to follow any advice given this book. For any products or services mentioned or suggested in this book, you should read all packaging and instructions, as no substance, natural or drug, can be guaranteed to work in everyone. Information and statements regarding dietary supplements, products or services mentioned in this book many not have been evaluated by the Food and Drug Administration and are not intended to diagnose, treat, cure, or prevent any disease. Never disregard or delay in seeking professional medical advice because of something you have read in this book.

Nothing that you read in this book should be regarded as medical or health advice. If you do anything recommended in this book, without the supervision of a licensed medical doctor, you do so at your own risk. Not recommended for persons with any health related condition unless supervised by a qualified health practitioner.

Because there is always some risk involved in any health-related program, the Author, Publisher and contributors assume no responsibility for any adverse effects or consequences resulting from the use of any suggested preparations or procedures described in any of the books or other written materials associated with the website FitnessThroughFasting.com. The author reserves the right to alter and update his opinions based on new conditions at any time.

Dedication

This series of books are dedicated to my mother Sonia Noemi, without whom I would not even be alive today. I love you mom. Thank you for never losing faith in me and supporting me, even when everything seemed hopeless and everyone else had given up on me. I owe you everything. I could collect all of the precious stones on this earth and lay them on your lap, and even still, I would not even come close to giving back to you all that you have given me.

Chapter 1:
Time for Breakthrough

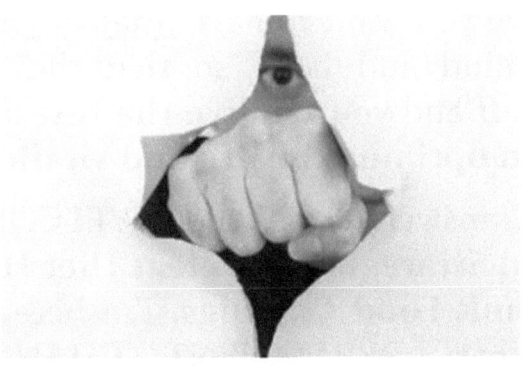

According to Dictionary.com, the word *"permanent"* means *"intended to exist or function for a long, indefinite period without regard to unforeseeable conditions; Long-lasting or nonfading."* In other words, whether it is raining, or whether it is sunny – whether things are going well or not so well, whether it feels good or it is difficult... no matter what is seen, felt or heard – one factor always remains:

What is **PERMANENT** <u>stays</u> the same. **NOTHING** moves it from its state of permanence. The quote by Dr. Joel Fuhrman is right on the money.

"You can't permanently change your health unless you permanently change your life."

My question to you is: do you want the word "<u>permanent</u>" to describe your weight loss? Do you want to have <u>total victory</u> over your mind and body so that the weight **stays off** and you can **live the rest of your days in optimum health and vitality?**

If you answered yes, then **WELCOME** to **Mental Strategies to Defeat Diet Hunger and Junk Food Cravings.** I'm here to tell you that: **PERMANENT CHANGE** is possible! Some years ago, I was 100 pounds overweight, trapped by overeating, isolated, depressed and suicidal. But I lost the weight and have **<u>NOT</u>** put it back on. That's what this volume is all about. Showing you mental techniques that will help you stick to your diet so that you, too, can achieve the same results.

And I have discovered that, as far as weight loss is concerned, *'the mind'* is what makes the difference between success and failure. Thoughts and emotions will attempt to lead you astray (*at first*). If you have tried to lose weight in the past and not made it, perhaps you understand what I'm talking about.

One moment you're super motivated and optimistic, then five minutes later, something happens and you feel weak, vulnerable and ready to call it quits. Yesterday you were able to easily say 'No' when the cravings (*or hunger*) came. Today, however, your resolve seems to have evaporated and, before you know it, *Whammo!* that pizza, donut (*or whatever*) is in your mouth again. Then, after the food is eaten, come the *horsemen of demoralization, condemnation, guilt and shame.* I was intimately familiar with this process and know just how devastating it can be to morale and overall self-esteem.

Why does it happen? If, in our heart of hearts, we truly want to lose weight and improve our health, why is it so easy to fall and return to poor eating and/or overeating? That is a very important question to answer because our lives and health depend on it. Weight loss is not a little game that we can take lightly. If you are more than twenty pounds overweight, or if you find yourself **yo-yoing** (*losing weight and regaining it over and over*), then the time has come to solve the problem. You owe it to yourself; and your loved ones will immensely benefit from your success. If I can do it, then by all means you can as well.

You can read my story (*as well as learn more ways to overcome overeating*) in my book **Binge Free (Triumph over Binge Eating) Confessions of a Former Food Addict**. The key to victory, I have found, has to do with developing a series of **strong mental techniques** that can shoot down the temptation, cravings and negative emotions that invite you to end the diet and/or eat in excess.

Worth the Initial Discomfort

It is important to note, however, that losing weight, and then working to keep it off, is not an overnight process. It can, as a matter of fact, be quite tough and challenging - especially during the first few months.

But, one thing is certain: The freedom that you can achieve is beyond description. So whatever initial discomfort you may have to go through now is **MORE** than worth it, trust me. Be encouraged and press toward the finish line without wavering.

About This Book

The first part of this book will focus on setting a strong foundation for weight loss. You will be asked to answer 20 key questions related to your weight loss goals. The questions are designed to give you an anchor that can hold you in place when temptation and/or cravings come. This part of the process is extremely important because you will put in writing the *'reasons'* why it is important for you to lose weight and improve your health.

Most of us usually know in our minds what these reasons are. However, when the temptation comes, the *'head knowledge'* is often insufficient to counteract the urge to stray. So it is of crucial importance to have this information in writing so that you can view it and *'remind yourself'* whenever you feel vulnerable. If you really want to achieve long-term weight loss, it is imperative to take the time to do this.

If you cut corners and skip the assignment, you may not be prepared to remain standing amidst a storm. It wasn't until I spent the time and worked on these questions to the very best of my ability that

I found lasting strength to stay the course and achieve my goals.

In the second part of the book we will talk about the direct connection between time and our thoughts, feelings and behaviors. Over the years I have found that: *Failure to understand the direct connection between the inner world of thought and emotion, with the external realm of behavior and time is a key reason why people lose weight but cannot keep it off.* Let me explain.

Chapter 2:
Trapped in Time

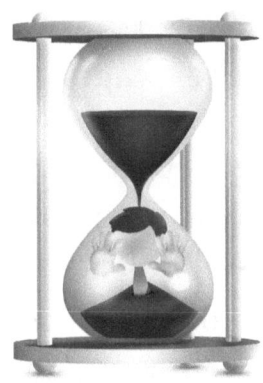

One of the **MOST COMMON** reasons why many people lose weight only to relapse into binging and/or destructive eating is that they allow their minds to use <u>TIME</u> to trap them into negative emotions and impulsive behavior.

In dozens of persons I have spoken to and/or coached over the years, the common answer to *"Why did you relapse"* is:

"I was convinced this [feeling, thought, discomfort] was going to last forever. Time was crawling and I became desperate! So I started eating, eating and eating. Next thing I know, I was binging again and felt horrible!"

Perhaps that statement is one you can relate to. It amazed me that these individuals – *none of who ever met (and even lived in different states and countries)* - came up with nearly identical answers as to **why they fell off the wagon**. Remarkably, I looked at many of my own weight loss journals from years past and found the <u>same</u> pattern! It was exciting because I saw that I was on to something that could help others.

A huge number of my journal entries were filled with complaints of *"how slow <u>time</u> was passing"*, *"how little weight I was losing"*, or – one of the worst – *"the huge amount of <u>time</u> it was going to take to reach my goal."* These entries were often accompanied with reasons as to why it was *"probably better to break the diet and try again <u>later</u>."* I was, in essence, <u>trapped in time</u>.

When we feel trapped, the usual response is to find a way to break free, right? Can you guess what that *"breaking free"* means during weight loss? Yep, it means straying from the diet – **often with a sense of urgency and even desperation**. Why? Because we are misled by the mind into believing that what we are feeling *(hunger* *pains, detox symptoms, irritability)* will not **EVER** pass **UNLESS** *"immediate remedial action is taken." "Better eat everything in sight, NOW!"* the mind says. *"Get back to safety; forget all this business about weight loss. It's impossible!"* The trap has been laid. You are now in danger of relapse. But the so called *"safety"* that the mind lures you towards ends up being <u>no safety at all</u>.

Instead – *in many cases* – the *"perceived act of safety"* culminates in **disorderly eating and all of the resulting disgust, shame and self-hatred that come with it**. It is a mental juggernaut that traps millions into a lifetime of obesity and sickness because, *unaware of this sinister mental snare*, they succumb time and again and stray from the path. In which ways has this *'time trap'* affected your own weight loss efforts? Do you feel like losing weight will take forever? That everything is happening too slowly?

And, if you have tried to lose weight and relapsed, did you fall off because you felt you couldn't hold on for another minute? These are all very common reasons. If this has happened to you, don't feel bad. The good news is that there <u>IS</u> a way to overcome moments of temptation, get through them and cross the finish line. Now let's move directly into the foundation phase. Later on, we will return to the time-trap and I will give you specific strategies that will help you to overcome.

Chapter 3:

The Road Less Travelled

The road you have begun to travel is certainly not an easy one. Any process of change is difficult, otherwise everyone would do it. If you are truly serious about losing weight and getting your health back on track, you are in the minority.

The pressures of modern life cause many of us to fall by the wayside with bad eating habits, destructive addictions and even downright laziness or apathy. *"Screw it"* was my motto for many years. It almost led me to my grave. I dove to depths of sickness and obesity beyond anything that I could have imagined. That's why I know that losing weight and keeping it off is a challenge. But it can be done.

It must be done.

Why should we live underneath our maximum potential? We know when we can do better; and it is our obligation to strive for optimum health. So I hope and pray that you are ready to take action and press on until you reach your goal. Honestly, you really don't have a choice. This is your life, and you should make it the very best that you can. I may not know you personally, but through these words I will pour out all that I have learned over the past 13 years as it relates to **weight loss and the mind**.

Chapter 4:

Weight Loss and the Mind

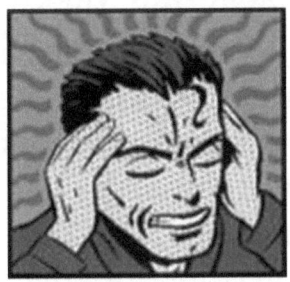

If you do a web search on *weight loss*, you will be bombarded with thousands upon thousands of pages on diets and diet supplements and pills. It all seems to be about *the outside*. Granted, weight loss <u>IS</u> about external results.

Nonetheless, I have discovered (*through bitter experience*) that simply working on the outside, in most cases, is not enough. If the mind is filled with bad habits, out-of-control emotions and other types of negativity, those patterns will - *in the end*- make us *fat* again. This is true whether the person is morbidly obese, overweight or just a bit chubby.

Our body weight, in essence, is directly linked to our thoughts, emotions and behaviors. I don't recall ever being chased down by a cheeseburger with legs, tackled to the ground and then having the burger force itself down my throat. No. It was always <u>me</u> who thought about the burger, craved the burger, drove to the burger joint, stood in line, ordered the sucker, paid for it and then inhaled it in the car without even leaving the parking lot. This happened to me over and over for decades. Then I realized that, in truth, the cheeseburger wasn't the problem.

Rather, it was my <u>lack of control</u>. If I could learn to master the thinking and behaviors that came **BEFORE** I ate the cheeseburger *(or any other type of unhealthy food), then I would be able to walk through the temptation and/or cravings <u>without</u> stuffing myself. The negative consequences could be completely avoided. That realization was hard to swallow at first (no pun intended). However, it also gave me a lot of hope because, for the first time in many years, I* ***started to see a way out of my dilemma.***

My Nightmare Experience
The toughest part of dieting, in my opinion, isn't hunger and cravings; it is **The Mental**

Battle. If you have been overweight and/or unhealthy for a long time, then you may experience some mental resistance when you first cut calories. You probably already know that by now. Some of this resistance may manifest itself in unpleasant thoughts, emotions and even vivid dreams.

When I did my first 40-day water fast, I was amidst was a very difficult period in my life. I was physically sick from a liver condition, was severely overweight and was stricken by a lot of emotional problems. Isolation and self-pity ruled my existence. I knew little of enjoying life; I was bitter, angry and simply wanted to die.

Cutting calories through fasting sent my mind into a state of immediate revolt. The second night of the fast, I started having vivid nightmares about demons and all kinds of weird things. At one point it felt as though I had left my body and was travelling around the world, floating in the air and observing people walking to and fro.

Strangers would approach me, smiling and offering all types of sugary and fattening foods. *Pastries and donuts have always been my primary triggers*. I was asleep, but my mind was wide awake. Being somehow conscious that I was fasting, I thanked the strangers for their offers but declined to take the junk food. Then, to my horror, their faces became deformed and evil, with fangs, claws and black hair that covered their entire bodies. Apparently enraged by my refusal to eat, some of these demons began to puncture my thighs, arms and legs with spikes. I could see the spikes impaling my legs, although I felt no pain. I tried to scream but found that I couldn't speak.

After God knows how long, I finally woke up drenched in sweat and shaking like a leaf. I was so scared that I couldn't go back to sleep that night. Instead, I wrote about the experience in my journal. After thinking about it long and hard, I concluded that the nightmare was a direct result of the calorie restriction. In my opinion, it was a manifestation of the destructive food addiction that controlled my life and did not wish to let go.

Up to that point, food had always been my drug of choice. I had never refused my stomach anything that it wanted. Gluttony and obesity were my lot. Then suddenly, there I was fasting and depriving the body of all of the junk that it always demanded. My mind and body went into shock! Still, it was absolutely necessary. If a person does not stop lighting cigarettes, he or she cannot stop smoking, right? By the same token, I had to stop eating "*completely*" for a season and allow my mind and body to "*withdraw*" from my addiction to junk food, particularly sugars and fat.

Although the dream scared me (*a lot*) at first, in the end it strengthened my resolve; I refused to continue being controlled by binging, fear, self-hatred, insecurity, immaturity and lack of discipline.

I share this experience with you not to scare you, but to emphasize that the mental aspect of weight loss is very real. The good news is that the initial resistance doesn't last. The mind and body can kick and scream, but if you hang in there and don't give up, within a few weeks the symptoms wane and the weight loss process gets easier. Helping you to reach that breakthrough point is what this book is all about.

A quick note: Be careful. Others can also

sabotage your progress if you let them. I know a gentleman who was trying to lose weight with all of his heart; he was 200 pounds overweight and had just been diagnosed with diabetes. He started the process wonderfully. However, his family members *(who were also obese)* began to constantly offer him junk food and fill the house with cakes and pastries. He eventually relapsed and, last time I saw him, he had gained another 50 pounds and looked terribly ill. I was so angry that I wanted to punch his brother in the face for not supporting his own flesh and blood.

Some people, for one reason or another, won't be happy that you want to improve your life and health.

Keep your eyes and ears peeled for such individuals and make every effort to stay away from them.

Only disclose your weight loss plans to people that you trust and know won't try to sabotage your efforts or fill you with unwanted advice, wisecracks and other nuisance comments.

Chapter 5:

Discarding the Negativity

Rome was not built in a day - but it **WAS** built. No matter how hopeless *(or not)* you may feel, I want you to collect all negativity and throw it in the trash. Many people that I talk to who are overweight (*or have struggled to lose weight*) are in the habit of being very harsh with themselves. They are filled with self-loathing, self-pity and bitterness. They feel like *losers* because of their inability to stick to a weight loss program. To be sure, oftentimes these emotions stem from deep-seated issues. But in most cases, the negativity can be interrupted by filling the mind with positive reasons to hang on.

If you berate yourself for not having reached your goals, or for having tried many times and not succeeded, the time has arrived to **halt the pessimism and find a better way**. That is my primary objective; to help you find a way that works, a system that can help you to <u>overcome obstacles</u> so that you can reach the finish line. But you have to be willing to do the work. I don't want you to simply glance over the material, set it aside and continue being fat, unhappy and unhealthy. I want you to produce measureable results. I want you to take strides toward your ultimate weight loss goals. If you are prepared to do the work, then we are halfway there.

Life is too darn short.

There is no time to waste. I lived the misery and pain that comes from allowing apathy to take over. One moment I was 17 years old with my whole life in front of me, then, next thing I knew, I was 35, obese, alone, suicidal and hopeless. I knew that unless I took whatever action was needed, I would be dead within a few years.

Here's the bottom line:

NOT taking action is not an option. Set aside all of your mental reservations and dive into this work with all of your might. You will be amazed at the results. Let's get started.

Chapter 6:
Setting the Foundation

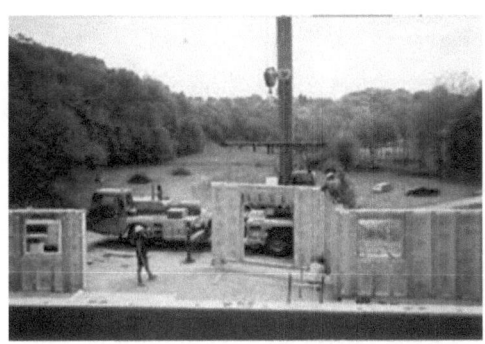

Any contractor will tell you that if a structure is built on a weak foundation, it will collapse. That is common sense. In this case, the foundation is simply this:

Putting in writing, in explicit detail, the specific reasons why you want to lose weight, and what impact reaching *(or not reaching)* your goal will have on your life.

Motivation is directly linked to our thoughts, feelings and behaviors. Nevertheless, as I said before, simply *thinking* about why you want to lose weight is a waste of time. The mind is way too complex. Life is full of pressures; it is easy to *forget* our goals at any given moment. You can start the weight loss process with the best of intentions, but when life gets in the way, you're going to need a lot more than positive intent.

A bad day at work, a traffic jam, an argument... any of these *(and others)* can – *in an instant* - be reason enough to gorge and break the diet. When we don't feel well and all looks bleak, we need something to bring us back to center.

For me, this meant rolling up my sleeves and taking stock of my life. I had to write about what was <u>important to me</u>. *Until I started to address the inner world of thoughts and emotions, I kept regaining every last pound I lost.* Then I discovered something that totally changed my attitude and perspective: Successful weight loss is about *mental focus*. Those two words are the key.

You need sufficiently-strong reasons IN WRITING so that, when the winds of temptation (or just stress) come, you can return to the reasons and remind yourself why it is important to get through that particular moment WITHOUT breaking the diet.

Read that last sentence a few times until you can fully internalize what it is saying. Armed with this realization, I started to put together a series of questions that forced me to confront the mental habits and behaviors that kept me from losing **ALL** of the weight. In a period of 18 months, I went from weighing 290 pounds to 195. Over the past ten years, my weight has fluctuated between *195 and 205* pounds; I have remained healthy and trim.

Coincidence?

I don't think so. I certainly am not stronger than you or have any special abilities. In fact, I was a total basket case when it came to food; I had the willpower of a gnat. At the site (*or thought*) of a donut, pastry, slice of pizza or cake, I would immediately start to salivate. Within seconds I was stuffing my face; diet and weight loss be dammed.

What made the difference was that, after years of misery and failure, I discovered a strategy that worked. You no longer have to spend years in the frustrating and painful see-saw of weight loss/weight gain. Change effected on the **INSIDE** gives permanency to what we do on the *OUTSIDE*.

While certainly not a conclusive system to deal with difficult issues as binging and overeating, the *questions* method outlined below is one that placed me in a position of <u>willingness to change.</u>

Having the *willingness to change* was a huge breakthrough for me because, for years, I was trapped in a very destructive action/reaction cycle that kept me toxic, overweight and highly disillusioned with life.

Chapter 6:

The Weight Loss Anchor

Your task is to answer each of these questions with the most gut-wrenching honesty that you can muster. *So here's what I need for you to do*: Buy a nice journal - one that represents you. In it, you will lay the foundation using the questions below as a guide.

Don't just start writing all of this in any *scratch* sheet of paper or used notebook. This is your future here! Give it some dignity and use a brand new journal, representing a new beginning in your life. Moreover, **take some quiet time to do this work**. Turn off the TV and the phone. Go somewhere where you won't be disturbed. You don't necessarily have to do them all at once. If you do, awesome. But these questions are designed to make you think, and to keep you thinking. So they're not just there to be answered once and 'I'm done.' The power of what you are doing lies in <u>continuity</u>: adding to it more and more as answers come to you day by day.

My suggestion is that you take your new journal with you wherever you go and continue to look at the questions and add to the answers whenever you have a free moment. I actually have like ten journals filled with answers to these questions. This has happened over a period of years, of course. But I think you get what I am trying to say; this is an ongoing task.

The more thorough you are with the answers, and the more explicit you are... the stronger a foundation you will have when moments of weakness come and you get the urge to give in, or give up.

Alright, enough blabbing... let's get to it.

Chapter 7:

Powerful Questions

1. Why do I eat when I know I should not?

In other words, what are the thoughts and feelings that you usually have when you binge, nibble, eat between meals and/or or overeat?

(Fear, Boredom, Anxiety, Depression, a feeling of impending doom etc.)

Take your time and be specific. In this question it is of supreme importance for you to meditate on your behavior as it relates to food. It may take a few minutes before you begin to identify the reasons. That's fine.

Don't rush. I have found that in **EVERY** case of overeating, nibbling or breaking a diet, a series of thoughts, feelings or external circumstances preceded the actual eating. For some people, overeating has become an <u>automatic loop</u>.

They are always reacting to thoughts, feelings and events without even realizing it. If you have never taken a close look at your eating behaviors, all of this may be a bit confusing and daunting. Push through it and move on. It will get easier over time and you will gain tremendous insight into your behaviors.

2. Does binging, nibbling and/or overeating provide a permanent solution to these thoughts and feelings?

In other words, are these compulsive actions producing *"better"* results in my life? This was the question that really did it for me so many years ago. *I realized that I was constantly eating in response to what happened outside as well as inside.*

However, no matter how much I ate, my life only got worse. It hit me like a ton of bricks: This eating equation did not work. Eating, giving in to cravings etc., did <u>not</u> improve anything in my life or '*solve*' the troubling thoughts and feelings. Rather, eating made everything worse. Meditate closely on your own eating behavior. Be honest with yourself. Has '*eating at your feelings and life circumstances*' made anything better?

3. Why do you feel that you can't help yourself? Is there a sense of impending doom or emotional nakedness that food helps you cover up?

Elaborate. This is a continuation of the previous question. Peel the layers of the onion and keep going deeper into your mind and heart. Trust me, if you are thorough and honest, a lot of stuff will begin to emerge that, possibly, you did not even know was there.

4. For how long does the relief last when you give in? What physical and mental outcomes does this behavior produce?

Weight Gain, Deteriorated Health etc. There was always a *'pay off'* for me to overeat, eat between meals and/or binge. There was a sense of <u>immediate gratification</u> that promised to give me relief from what I was feeling. Even if what I was feeling was mundane like boredom, there was a payoff nonetheless. However, the consequences of my actions were always negative.

I was bloated, felt tired all the time, had constant *(and violent)* sugar cravings, trouble sleeping, etc. In this question, I want you to identify what payoff you get when you overeat, eat between meals or give in to temptation.

5. At what point does the *'pleasure'* dissipate and you start to feel bad *(emotionally or physically)* about what you did?

(Example: Guilty, Ashamed, Hating Myself, Bloated, Tired, Nauseous etc.). I know this question is quite compound, so take your time and let it all sink in before you start

answering it.

6. What are the specific trigger foods and/or beverages that I gravitate to?

Mention them specifically; donuts, pizza, soft drinks, cake etc. Do you buy them and keep them in the house? Order them by phone, the Internet?

For this question, I suggest that you take some time and take **a thorough food inventory**, with emphasis on the foods that you tend to abuse or have a special weakness towards. Name the usual suspects, but take time to think of others who may not be as obvious.

7. How do I feel once I give in to the urge to eat these foods?

Disgusted, Depressed, Angry etc. Be very personal and specific. This question is a continuation of number 5. However, here I want you to associate the feelings directly with the trigger foods.

(Example: When I give in and eat the cheeseburger or nibble on candy between meals, I feel like crap because I have undone some of my progress, am back to the same trap etc.).

The importance of this question is immense because I want you to realize more and more the destructive power that these foods have on your long-term goals. Even though there is dubious pleasure on the short-term, it really isn't worth it in view of the long-term chaos that they cause, what do you think?

8. Am I willing to admit that my relationship with food and eating is therefore faulty and in need of revision?

If yes, explain how. *(Example: because overeating will never cover feelings, provide real fulfillment etc. Because I am overweight and unhappy and my eating is making everything worse and worse.)*

9. Can I see that my relationship with food and eating is based on a faulty

equation that just makes everything worse?

If yes, explain how. *(Example: because no matter how much I eat, I keep feeling down. Because months and years go by and I am still overweight, unhappy and getting worse etc.)*

10. What will happen short-term if I DO NOT resist these urges and continue down the same road?

In other words, over the coming days, weeks and months, how is your life going to be and how are you going to feel if you do nothing and allow these habits to go on unbridled? Be as explicit as you can.

11. What is the ultimate long-term consequence that I will pay if I do not take action NOW to change these thinking and behavior patterns as they relate to food and eating? Be explicit!

12. What will my life be like in 10 years if I do not take action now?

Mentally, physically, socially, spiritually etc. Remember *The Ghost of Christmas Future from A Christmas Carroll*? Well, this is it. Use it! Dig deep into your heart and mind and look at yourself 10, 15 years from now **NOT** having done anything about your weight and health.

What do you see? How do you look? How do you feel? How is your health?

13. Am I willing to pay these negative consequences? Why not?

Be detailed. *(Example: because I want to be around for my children, travel abroad, get married, continue to advance in my career, be prosperous, have a lavish life, not develop a chronic illness etc.).*

As I said earlier, it is important that you take your time and come up with strong answers. If you just jot down a one-sentence response without giving the questions deep and serious thought, then you are wasting your time.

These questions are meant to strip your soul bare and force you to cough up deep-seated thoughts and feelings.

That is not to say that initially you may only come up with one sentence. That is fine. But don't give up... keep meditating on the question and continue to probe your mind and heart for answers. Believe me, they are there!

14. How would I feel if I STOPPED feeding into these food impulses and began to say said NO?

(Example: Empowered, Good about myself, Hopeful etc.). Why would I feel these positive feelings? *(Example: Because I will have resisted something that harms me, because I will have gained self-esteem, because I would start to feel lighter, healthier, more attractive etc.).*

This is the pivotal point where you can begin to see that <u>NOT</u> giving in to these urges is the ONLY way to true happiness and satisfaction. Giving in may feel good at that immediate moment, but saying no and delaying gratification is the road to the ultimate victory that you seek.

15. What would happen if I resist these urges to eat? Do I feel like I would collapse or die? Can I recognize that these are lies?

Explain the reasons the mind gives you as to why resisting these food impulses is *'too hard'* or even *'impossible.' (Example: When I am tempted, I feel like I simply cannot resist. The cravings are just too strong)*.

Can you internalize the reality that this is a lie? That you are **NOT** helpless? That you **CAN** get through it? *(Example: Resisting these cravings is NOT impossible because I will NOT die if I do not give in, etc.)*.

The key to this question is realizing that any short-term discomfort you may feel from resisting the food urges will pass, that you will not fall to pieces if you hold your ground.

As a matter of fact, I can tell you from

experience that cravings and temptations rarely last more than 30 minutes. Once they pass, the sense of satisfaction is amazing.

16. What is the ultimate truth for you?
(Example: I must change my impulsive eating and I must stop giving in to the cravings and food urges because otherwise I will never reach my goal, I will feel unhappy, I will feel unfulfilled, I risk illness etc.). In view of the answers to all of the previous questions, what conclusion have you reached?

17. What real choice do you have than to change?

Continuing to give in to hunger through binging, nibbling and/or compulsive eating is <u>not</u> the answer. It will never be the answer. It will never work. *Continuing to give in to binging, nibbling and/or compulsive overeating will always lead you to negative outcomes in your life.* Period.

18. Can you admit this to yourself and understand it?

Explain why you admit it and why you understand it. If you can admit to yourself that the status-quo doesn't work and that immediate change is imperative, and if you can write in detail the reasons why this is so, then you are on your way to some pretty dramatic changes in your food behaviors.

19. So this begs the question: **What is your choice going to be?**

(Example: My choice will be to do whatever it takes and go through whatever short-term discomfort I need to in order to overcome and reach my weight loss goals). Explain the *"why"* of your choice.

20. What are you willing to do to achieve the life that you deserve?

Here we reinforce the previous question with detail of what you are now prepared to do to reach your goals. *(Example: I am willing to walk through the urge to binge, feel the pain of not doing so, deal with hunger pains directly even if I want to give up and give in)* This last answer is important because it provides powerful reasons for you

to hang on to when you feel like giving up.
So be detailed!

Chapter 8:

How to Use the Journal

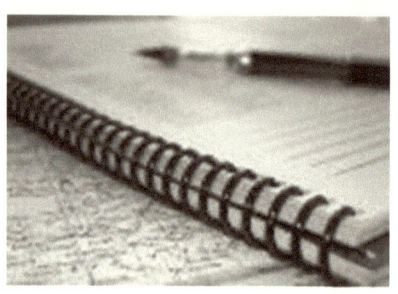

Don't allow the amount of questions to overwhelm you. Just start writing and let the answers come out as they may. At first you may only come up with short answers.

But I guarantee you that, if you persist, you will start to go deeper and deeper. Truly, you will be amazed at some of the stuff that will come out. Several times I wrote things that left me saying, *huh?* Where the heck did this come from?

Well, it was there all along. I was reacting to it and allowing it to thwart my efforts, but was largely unaware of it. **So persistence is key!** Some people write me and tell me: *"Robert, I just don't like to write."*

My answer is always the same: *"Too bad. Get over it and do it anyway."* If you are dragging your feet or feeling apathetic about doing the work, then I have to question your commitment to change. Look, it is never easy to push forward at first.

There is a lot of <u>inner resistance</u> that we have to overcome initially. But **it won't get any easier if we do nothing about it**. It will fester and get worse. So make sure to spend time daily with this journal. However, don't just write on it and then slip it in a drawer. <u>Take it with you wherever you go</u>. Keep it nearby and add to it whenever you have a moment. But you **MUST** have the journal with you at all times.

You never know when a craving or urge to give in will come. It is at that moment that you need to pull it out and start reading it. *Here's what happens*: The craving and/or urge to break the diet comes around. I am having a bad day, traffic is a nightmare, my boss is being a jerk, the children are misbehaving and on and on. At that moment, I don't give a hoot about anything. I just want relief, the trigger food is there and, honestly, I feel totally justified in eating it because life is feeling very uncomfortable. In that instant, if all you have are reasons *floating in your mind*, I can assure you that - *in many cases* - it won't be enough.

You have to pull out the journal and start reading it right away to interrupt the craving and remind yourself why sticking to the diet is far more important than any fleeting emotion or annoyance that may be going on.

It's really that simple. That's why I call this the *weight loss anchor*. It is easy to stray during weight loss. We need something to hold us in place, and the journal will do exactly that **if you put it to use**. What I notice is that, no matter how harsh the craving, it pretty much evaporates once I get into the journal and start reading the answers.

Often I take that moment to expand on one of the questions, or simply write down what I am feeling. Within 15 minutes it's all forgotten and I've moved on with my day without succumbing to the craving and sabotaging my goals. Just do it. There aren't any 'yeah buts' here that have any validity. If you are fed up with failing to lose weight and keeping it off, then taking this action on an ongoing basis will help to keep you grounded. If it worked for such a hopeless case as myself, then I have no doubt that it can do the same for you.

Chapter 9:

Confronting the Food Urges

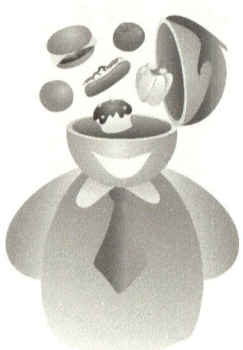

I realize that I have bombarded the living daylights out of you. I know that this is a lot and that it can be hard work. That is why most people don't do it and then fail. If you answered these questions honestly, the end conclusion will look something like this:

If you want to have a life of health and fulfillment, then you really DO NOT have a choice. You MUST confront hunger and cravings NOW and find a better way to live.

The most important part of this assignment is that of *unmasking* the thoughts, feelings and urges that lead you to give in and not stick to your diet. Unmasking the reality that these aren't *innocent, harmless little impulses.* Rather, they are destructive *(yet subtle)* forces that, if left unchecked, lead to only negative physical and emotional consequences.

You don't have to be obese or in danger of sickness for this to be true. Even if you only have a few pounds to lose, you have goals and they are important. Not reaching them will still cause dissatisfaction and a sense that you could have done better. And, to me, there is **NO** excuse for settling for less than the best in health and quality of life. So I encourage you to take out your journal and, *over the coming days and weeks,* answer **ALL** of the questions.

Take as much time as you need. **BUT DO IT!** This technique will be indispensable as you move forward with your weight loss program; it will give you enhanced clarity and motivation to go all the way. I can tell you from experience that negative/obsessive thoughts, feelings and behaviors are attached to lifestyle and eating habits. Who has not eaten for emotional comfort?

Note: This **IS NOT** to say that, as human beings, we do not have moments of weakness. If I occasionally eat a slice of apple pie, there's no need to put myself down or feel bad.

What **I AM** saying is that unhealthy food impulses that have been with us for years *(and produce nothing but unhappiness and failure)* must be confronted and expelled – by force if necessary. When I started to do this on a regular basis, I found that *the desperation to overeat* and binge began to subside. I could be struck with a craving for pastries *(or anything else)* and, instead of blindingly giving in, I'd pull out the journal and reinforce the reasons why it was important to say **NO**.

While in the past I would never last more than a few weeks on any diet, months began to go by and I was sticking to my guns! It was truly miraculous. I tapped into a powerful inner truth and was thus able to deal with the cravings, thoughts and feelings directly - **without having to reach for anything outside of myself to give me an artificial sense of wellbeing**. The life-long sugar addiction was broken because I abstained long enough for the body to detoxify, thus wiping out the terrible cravings that made me a slave for so many years. Here's the message to you:

The more time you spend on these questions, the more you will benefit.

It's a powerful tool that will lead you to the breakthrough you seek! How you use them is up to you. But use them you must!

About Depression: I am not a psychiatrist, and neither do I intend to provide medical or mental health advice. But I **AM** familiar with depression and know the devastation and literal **HELL** it can put a person through if left unchecked.

Depression was definitely one of the reasons why I had a marked tendency to isolate and eat compulsively. While losing weight and getting healthy will have a tremendous impact on how you feel, I strongly urge you to seek professional help if you feel this is a problem. You do not have to suffer and certainly deserve to be happy!

A Final Word: The questions I have shared with you are intended to get you thinking. I want you to realize that it **IS** possible to make long-lasting changes in your weight and health. If you can acquire a *heart-felt* willingness to change and set aside your prejudices and pre-conceived notions *(we all have them to one degree or another)*, then you're definitely on your way.

Now, let's go deeper and look at specific mental tricks and techniques you can use to avert temptation and stick to your diet.

Chapter 10:

The Powerful Present

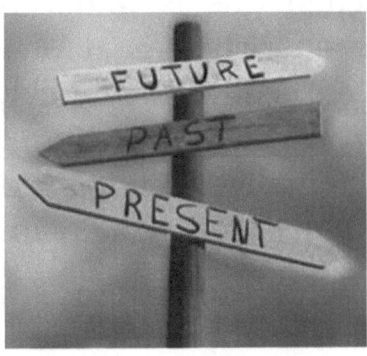

A very powerful antidote to the vicious and crippling cycle of weight loss and then binging and gaining it back over and over is this: Learning to *"forcefully"* bring the mind to the immediate present when the body, thoughts and emotions beckon you to give up.

It's important to realize that weight loss (and any change in eating habits) will bring most (if not all) of our human weaknesses to the surface.

This can manifest itself in all types of negative emotions, particularly in the first days of a calorie restriction program.

You may feel angry one moment, and then find yourself weeping the next. You can go from total and absolute motivation, to wanting to throw in the towel in a matter of minutes. When one is under this type of assault, the cherished goal of weight loss and improved health can quickly become a secondary, far-away illusion. At that moment, actually staying the course indefinitely will seem virtually impossible.

The mind will attempt to swallow your dreams and trap them in time – all of this fueled by your very thoughts, feelings and cravings. Ultimate self-sabotage; indivisible devastation! And, to end *the suffering*, the mind will invite you to eat whatever food is in sight – regardless of how toxic and destructive.

In fact, the more toxic and destructive the better because *"you will receive more comfort,"* the mind will say. I was struck down by this monster over and over for more than 20 years. We must expose the enemy in order to effectively stand against it. In this case, the 'enemy' becomes *a warped concept of time that throws our senses (sight, sound, smell) into overload and impulsive (and counterproductive) action.*

Ok ... stop for a moment and <u>take a deep breath</u>. That was a lot of information in a few short paragraphs. Are you with me so far?

What I have described is **an attack on everything that you wish to accomplish**. It is the very foe in our minds that will try to steal our hopes and dreams! The most baffling part is that the assault is not carried out by an outside force; the prime and sole perpetrator is – <u>OUR MINDS</u>!

In The Present Tense

Much has been written about the power of the <u>present moment</u>. Authors like Eckhart Tolle and his renowned *Power of Now* series illustrate very clearly how our **false perception of time** can cause tremendous emotional hardship and long-term suffering.

My own interpretation of the *present moment* concept is this: Since the past is gone and the future does not exist, any long-term focus on them will usually create anxiety, sadness, anger, fear etc. Why? Because there is absolutely nothing that we can do about the past **OR** the future.

We have no power whatsoever to make time go by faster or to go back in time and relive a past era or moment of our lives. This is what Tolle refers to as *psychological time.* The past and future exist **ONLY** in our minds, nowhere else. They are but illusions and have little *(if anything)* to do with the actual present *(reality)*.

A good friend of mine who I will call Paul clearly illustrates how terrible this time trap can be. He suffers from severe binge-eating disorder and, as of the last time we spoke, was 200 pounds overweight. He always starts out strong with his weight loss program, but never lasts more than two weeks.

The reason for his chronic relapsing, he says, is that when time starts to pass, he remembers the great times he had in the 1980s and feels an overwhelming urge to *celebrate.* Even though I've tried to *'make him see'* the distortion in which he is caught, the *'celebration'* continues to this day. The antidote to this crippling *(and unproductive)* state of mind is nothing more and nothing less than **learning to live in**

the absolute present moment. Do you know why? Because <u>the present is eternity</u>. And harmful emotions based on the past and future cannot exist in the eternal now.

They are gobbled up in the same way that a black hole in space swallows gravity and even light. The present is freedom; and there's no other place to find it except in the here and now. To accomplish this, we must accept the fact that **we are totally powerless over anything else except the present**.

Therefore, wasting time thinking about the past and future will do nothing but <u>continue to contaminate the present</u>. That isn't to say that one cannot reminisce of good times, regress in order to identify and heal wounds, or even plan for the future.

Those are all productive ways to live a better *NOW*. However, when the thoughts of the past and future are constant, morbid and not part of any self-improvement effort, then we are *trapped in time* and in danger of acting impulsively as an effort to <u>soothe</u> the emotional pain.

Chapter 11

Escaping the 'Time Trap'

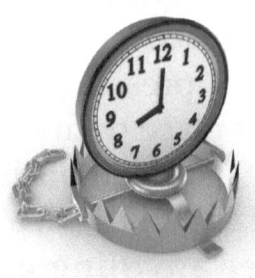

I invite you to read this volume several times until you can start to identify how this trickery operates in your own mind. It may take some time for you to notice it because it often takes place <u>under the level of consciousness</u>.

So now, let's look at a mental technique that has helped me to stay the course in moments of intense discomfort and temptation. First of all, when these difficult moments arise and you are tempted to stray from your diet, **STOP!** Bring all of your mental focus to the immediate present.

<u>Do this</u>:

*Look at your hands and feet and bring to your attention what you are doing and where you are at that particular time. Are you at the supermarket? At the office? At home? In the car? Are you driving? Walking? Working? Out with friends? Cooking for your family? Example: *"Ok, Robert – you are <u>NOW</u> at the supermarket walking down the cereal aisle.* <u>NOW</u> is the key word.

*Pause and focus your mind solely on what is happening at that moment. When other thoughts and feelings related to food, eating and giving up try to force their way through, push them back and look closely at what is happening around you.

Here's how you can wipe out the craving/desire to break the diet:

*Place Emphasis on Your Sense of Sound. I wrote this entry in my journal when I was hit by a massive craving for sugar while in a supermarket:

"I am NOW pushing a shopping cart with a squeaky wheel and listening to music playing over the loudspeaker. I can hear myself

walking; people are talking all around me; a baby is crying nearby; the cashier is asking for a price check etc." The key is to listen for any and all sounds within earshot. Go deep.

What sounds can you identify that you would normally not hear? Can you hear other people's footsteps? What about the air conditioner or other machinery? Try to discover as many *'new'* sounds as possible. Close your eyes if it helps. Trust me, there are **MANY** things going on around us that we barely ever see or hear. The deeper you go in your search for sound, the quicker the craving will dissolve.

But you can go even further.

Keeping the above two steps active in your mind, **tighten the mental reigns and start to visually peruse everything around you, in detail.** Here's another entry from my journal:

"The floor is gray; the shelves are painted beige; the man in front of me is wearing a black pair of pants with a blue sports jacket, argyle socks and two-toned shoes (anybody still dress like this?). I see people coming in and out of the store.

Go deep. Scan your surroundings and focus your sight in as much detail as possible.

Then you can combine both sight and sound and immerse yourself in every little detail that you can hear and see.

It never fails that, within a few minutes, I am feeling better and the craving has vanished. This strategy will require practice, especially if, like me, you have given in easily to hunger in the past. But the more you practice, the deeper you will go and the faster the cravings will disappear.

Chapter 12:

The Weapons of Sight and Sound

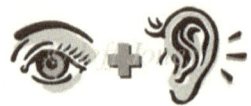

The strategy is to fill your sight and hearing with as much detail as possible of what is happening in the <u>IMMEDIATE PRESENT</u>. At first you may feel silly. The mind may tell you that you are wasting your time. That it doesn't work.

The mind may press you with more acute hunger and/or irritability – you may feel hopeless. It is at that precise moment that you must take the battle directly to the mind and persist with the exercise. If you give yourself <u>COMPLETELY</u> to the technique, you will find yourself – *over a period of 5 to 15 minutes* – immersing your mental energy into **NOW**.

And the <u>NOW</u>, without fail, will <u>ALWAYS</u> consume these attacks! It is guaranteed. There is <u>ZERO</u> opportunity for these imps to survive when the immediate present is summoned.

Lost In Thought

The problem with most of us is that we are lost in our own thoughts and hardly ever stop to look at what is happening around us. I will give you a good example from **MY** own life: I drove by a flea market daily for three years and **NEVER** noticed it until a friend invited me to visit it. Another time I was trying to find a shoe-repair shop and did not realize there was one a block from my home. I had walked and driven by it constantly, **looking at it but not seeing it**.

Moreover, I lived in a house that was surrounded by beautiful lush trees, many of which were utilized by a variety of birds to breed and nest their young. Most mornings there were countless little birds singing outside my bedroom window. But, honestly, it **is very hard for me to remember ever listening!** If you asked me what the bird song sounded like I would **NOT** be able to tell you! I heard but did not listen.

I spent most of my waking moments trapped in the mind thinking about the past and/or future, barely taking a moment to see or hear the present moment.

Many people live their whole lives in this disempowering state. They are locked inside their own minds, constantly replaying scenarios of the past and future. This elicits unpleasant emotions that, in turn, lead to obsessive and compulsive behavior designed to "*medicate*" the pain.

Unfortunately, the obsessive/compulsive action brings only short-term relief. The behavior ends up becoming an overpowering monster capable of consuming a person's entire life via binging, overeating, nibbling, grazing, etc. This mental prison fueled my binging and overeating for many years.

I was always anxious, irritable and discontent, always reacting to the *lies and distortions* that the mind was feeding me.

In short, the *Time Trap Escape* reminds us to break away from the snare of constant thought. It teaches us step out of our minds frequently and just **be** by absorbing the sights and sounds of life. The discomfort associated during weight loss is minimized *(and even eliminated)* when one becomes adept at this simple *(yet extremely powerful)* exercise.

The soothing calm that comes over the entire body once the attack is over is amazing. It will help you to realize that the demands and loud voices within, ultimately, only have power over your actions if you let them. If you feel daring, I invite you to spend longer and longer periods of time each day in this state of *"present mindedness."*

The exercise is especially effective while one is dieting and/or making significant dietary changes. It is like doing **mental push-ups.** At first you may only be able to do five pushups, with much struggle and exertion. But, if you continue to train, in a short time you will be able to do more. The same is the case with the mind, my dear friend.

Practicing present moment focus has been my biggest ally. To focus exclusively on what is in front of me. This is difficult because most of us are accustomed to letting the mind wonder aimlessly like a wild horse without a bridle. Weight loss, therefore, goes beyond just eating less and working out. It places us face-to-face with our undisciplined thinking and impulsivity.

Calorie restriction disciplines the mind as well as the body.

But we must be willing to adopt new thinking strategies that can help us sustain the benefits. I learned after much trial and error that food was a mere symptom of my undisciplined/obsessive thinking.

Indeed, losing weight will help you to look and feel much better. But the benefits will not last unless you humbly commit yourself to reclaiming control over your mind. To this end, I invite you to also read my book **How to Lose Weight & Keep it Off by Reprogramming the Subconscious Mind** as well as **The Cravings Ninja** Assassin. Let's go deeper into this process of mental renovation/change.

Chapter 13:

Psychic Change

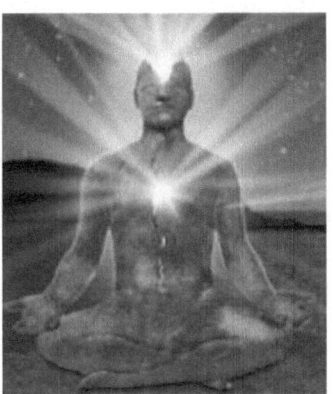

No matter where you are in your journey of heath-improvement, one constant factor I have seen over the years is this:

Permanent Weight Loss and Optimum Health Is Best Achieved through Internal Change in Thoughts and Attitudes.

I define the phrase psychic change as follows:

A revolution of the mind and spirit which leads an individual to a new way of thinking, behaving and sustaining personal freedom.

A psychic change will help you to maintain weight loss and health because you will learn to think, behave and live differently. And you will get closer to attaining it the measure that you start to confront the mental attacks and cravings that lead you to stray.

There are no words to describe the joy and peace that you will feel when a temptation comes up and you get through it without breaking the diet. It's like: *Wow! I can actually do this!* You will start to gain a mastery over your body and appetite that you thought was impossible. In most cases, the change comes gradually over a period of time, although there are some who experience it quickly and intensely.

What I am trying to tell you is this:

The discomfort that you go through during weight loss does not have to be viewed as a punishment or something negative. Certainly, it is uncomfortable, but the discomfort can actually lead you to higher levels of mental acuity and awareness; it will help you to develop 'mental muscles' to resist cravings and temptations. And these crucial muscles cannot be built any other way than through pressure. If you can reframe the weight loss process into this positive perspective, you will gain strength and not feel like you are walking through a trail of tears.

Let's take a look at a few more techniques you can incorporate into your mental weaponry.

Chapter 14:

Detox Breathing

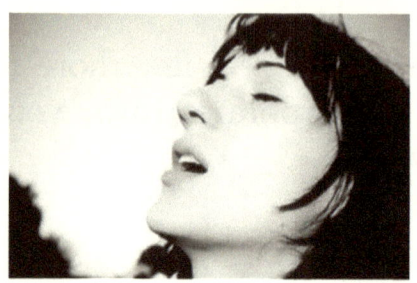

When tempted to give in, we must pull out every weapon in the arsenal. The *Time Trap Escape* will place you in a position of offense. Now, let's go a step further and continue the counterattack through what I call *Detox Breathing (DB)*. *DB* is one of the most important tools you can use to overcome cravings and temptation.

Breathing is the essence of life.

Without breathing there is no life. I am not talking about the typical *"breathe in, breathe out"* exercise that one associates with meditation or the 1985 movie *The Karate Kid*.

That type of breathing is indeed great and I

encourage you to practice it. *DB*, on the other hand, is comprised of **intense 10-minute breathing sessions designed to give you an immediate physical and mental boost**. I have found this *espresso shot* of oxygen to be amazingly beneficial in reducing mental negativity, hunger and detoxification symptoms. I use it constantly.

The problem is that many people have not learned how to breathe properly.

They do not realize that reduced oxygen intake causes them to be tired and lethargic; it slows the thought process and breeds depression and negativity. Indeed, you have tremendous life-giving power in your lungs.

One of the first things that I observe when I meet a personal coaching client is the person's breathing pattern. **Nearly 100% breathe shallow**. Very seldom – if ever – do people STOP and *practice the art of breathing*. The moment has come for you to start.

*Special Note: Do you snore? If so, you may suffer from a condition known as **Obstructive Sleep Apnea**. OSA can make this entire process TWICE as hard because your breathing is blocked while you sleep and* *the brain does not get enough oxygen. Not to mention that your body cannot fall into the deep sleep required for proper rest.*

So if you have been blamed for *cutting logs* and/or *roaring like a bear* then I encourage you to go see your doctor. He or she may send you for a sleep test to determine if you have this dangerous condition. If so, you may need to incorporate the use of a **Positive Airway Pressure Machine**. Weight loss will also help.

Detox Breathing in Practice

When a craving or temptation hits, do this: Immediately put to practice the *Time Trap Escape.* Find a place where you can be undisturbed for 10 minutes. Sit down and close your eyes.

Take the deepest breath that your lungs allow.

Breathe in until you cannot take in any more oxygen. Count the seconds as you inhale. Depending on the condition of your lungs, you will be able to count to five or 10. If you are unable to get to five ... don't worry. Your lung capacity will actually improve as you continue to practice *DB*.

Inhale and count simultaneously until your lungs are completely full. As you count, visualize that you are breathing in white, glowing, healing oxygen ... see the white air in your mind's eye. If you are not used to breathing deep, you may feel aches and pains on your back, chest and throat. Those aches will also disappear as you practice.

1) **Once you have inhaled as much air as the lungs permit, visualize the white, powerful oxygen navigating around your entire being**.

   Whatever number you reached during the inhalation, <u>multiply it times eight</u>. If, for example, the inhalation lasted seven seconds, multiply that times eight for a total of 56. Now hold your breath for the resulting amount of seconds, in this case 56 seconds. If you cannot reach the X8 goal, do the very best that you can. Build up to it.

2) **As you hold your breath, keep visualizing your body being filled with a white light representing the healing oxygen that you inhaled**.

   Observe as the white light covers your legs, arms, heart *(the seat of the emotions)* and ultimately - your brain. By the time you are halfway through the X8 count, visualize **your entire being engulfed by the white light**. At this point you may start to feel dizzy and experience a *head rush*. That is normal; your body may not be accustomed to receiving such a concentrated amount of oxygen.

Place all of your mental faculties into this simple visualization. Allow all other distracting thoughts to pass/ use the *Time Trap Escape* to focus on the present moment. Whatever is troubling you at the time ... whether it be negative thoughts, an emotion or just plain old fashioned hunger – **visualize them being covered and consumed by the white light**.

3) When the X8 count is completed, start to **SLOWLY** exhale out of your mouth.

Visualize the exhalation as black air containing everything that is disturbing you.

Take your time and *see* this dark, ugly air being expelled from your body, **taking with it all of the negativity and**

discomfort. You are free. Continue to exhale *slowly* and focus on the **black air** coming out of your mouth until the lungs are <u>COMPLETELY</u> empty. The exhalation process should take at least half of the time that it took to inhale.

As in the example above, if the X8 inhalation was 56 seconds, then the exhalation should take around 25 seconds. When exhaling, make sure to *blow out* every last bit of air from your lungs, as if you were putting out the candles in a birthday cake. The *black air* visualization should continue up to the very end.

Light and healing in – Darkness and discomfort out. Light and peace in – stress and anger out. Motivation and mental clarity in – hunger pains and detox symptoms out.

4) **Repeat the first three steps until you have given yourself a *break* of at least ten minutes.**

If you have more time, by all means continue. I usually try to do around five inhalations and exhalations per *DB* session. The longer you do it, the greater the benefit. However, I suggest that, at first, you do no more than three inhalation/exhalations until your body gets used to the exercise.

Some people have reported intense lightheadedness when doing this type of intense breathing. So take it easy and work your way up slowly. As you will discover, *DB* is very powerful. I have gone from imminent physical and emotional collapse to restored clarity and motivation with the aid of this simple technique, in combination with the *Time Trap Escape.*

At one point I almost broke a 120-day liquid fast out of anger and because I was craving a glazed donut. Ten minutes of *DB* saved the day. Doing it while driving *(with eyes open of course!)* is helpful. Rather than sitting in traffic annoyed, be productive and practice *DB*.

Breathing and Your Health

There are also specific health reasons to practice *DB*. The rhythmic motion of the lungs is very important to expel excess mucus, which can inhibit breathing.

Slow, deep breathing gets rid of carbon dioxide waste and takes in plenty of clean, fresh oxygen. Blood cells get the new, oxygen-rich air (white light) and the body expels the stale one (black air).

DB helps the body eliminate carbon dioxide much faster than shallow breathing. You'll not only be healthier, but you'll perform better, be less stressed and feel more relaxed.

This will help you immensely to handle hunger, cravings and the emotional see-saw incited by the lifestyle changes you are making.

Chapter 15:

Release the Serpent

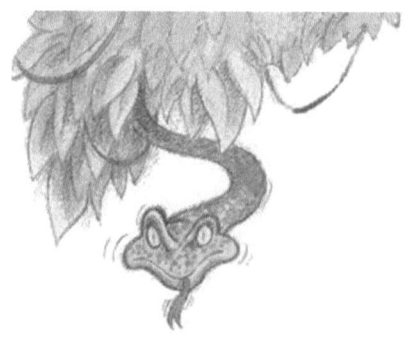

If you take the time to practice the *Time Trap Escape* in conjunction with *Detox Breathing (as well as regularly reading and writing on your journal)*, there will come a time when no temptation to eat will be able to overcome you. I know that this is a big promise, but it has proven true in my life over and over.

What is needed is commitment, practice and perseverance. But I want to go further and give you yet another tool that you can add to the arsenal, and that is what I call **Release the Serpent** *(RTS).*

As we have seen, the key to success in

weight loss, apart from diet and exercise, is proper use of the mind. *RTS* is a mental visualization that will help you eliminate *any thought or behavior that goes against what you are trying to accomplish.*

Done persistently, *RTS* (*together with the Time Trap Escape and Detox Breathing*) will give you strength, resolve and commitment to overcome hunger, cravings and uncomfortable emotions. I will illustrate how *RTS* works with an analogy.

A person handling a snake by the middle of its body complains of being constantly bitten. But this person refuses to let go of the serpent. Day after day the individual continues to handle the snake; day after day he or she is bitten. However, after one particularly nasty bite, this person makes a determined decision:

"I will no longer hold the snake mid-body. Instead, I will hold on to its tail!"

Let me ask you: Is this person any safer as a result of that decision? Indeed, he or she may have a *perceived sense* of safety. But, in reality, **the person is no better off**. Safety is an illusion because he or she is **STILL** holding the snake, albeit in a different place.

The person has <u>NOT</u> let go and is <u>still</u> in danger. No matter how careful this person is, he or she will likely be bitten again in a moment of vulnerability or distraction. So what is the solution? The only sure way to be safe would be to completely let go of the snake and walk away, <u>to no longer be in its presence or have any contact with it</u>.

The weight loss process is very similar.

The surest way to be successful is to let go of the serpent COMPLETELY and walk in the opposite direction.

This begs the question: What is the serpent?

The serpent represents the insidious mental arguments, suggestions and/or conversations that fuel any action and/or behavior that goes against your weight loss goals.

The *opposite direction* represents sticking to the diet in spite of the discomfort, continuing to move toward your goal without giving in to the mental chatter. Understand this: The serpent is <u>ALWAYS</u> in the mind.

That is where the battle rages.

It is the source! Hunger and physical symptoms will pass, but the serpent's endless arguments and suggestions can keep a person forever succumbing to actions and/or behaviors that destroy positive objectives, in this case long-term weight loss and health. I cannot tell you how many times I hear:

"Robert, I start out the day feeling very motivated, but then something happens and – bang! - I break the diet and am back to square one!"

If, however, you let go of the serpent *(completely)* and walk away from it, then the mental chatter is immediately silenced because **you're no longer in the snake's proximity**. Since the serpent isn't around anymore to entice you, you'll be less likely to stray.

No matter how uncomfortable the physical symptoms become, *RTS* will help you to weather the storm and press on. You will learn to face the discomfort and walk through it, **without giving in to temptation**. That was the biggest breakthrough that I could have ever experienced. After countless years of failure and disappointment, I suddenly had a winning perspective; I felt liberated.

With the serpent out of the picture, you can rest in an inner silence that will empower you. This vacuum of stillness will allow the mind to start working in your favor rather than as a constant saboteur. Your mental resources will be elevated to a much higher plane because the negative mental arguments will be invalidated.

Hunger and physical cravings come and go. But you can walk through them every time with the proper mental perspective. You are neither a victim nor a slave. You are a victor!

RTS gave me the key that unlocked the mental prison in which I had lived for nearly 25 years. Indeed, the amazing power behind this simple visualization never ceases to astonish me. And it can help you too! Here's how:

Release the Serpent in Action

When hunger, cravings and/or uncomfortable thoughts and emotions tempt you to break your diet, <u>DO THIS</u>:

*Visualize yourself holding a serpent by its tail. As we have already seen, the snake represents mental suggestions and arguments that invite you to abandon your weight loss program. It is an internal voice that is constantly presenting reasons, justifications and rationalizations why you should forget about losing weight and give in to temptation. The first step is for you to identify the thought and/or arguments.

*Keep it simple and to-the-point. In my case, the most common argument is:

"Robert, go eat a donut! You can't do this anymore. You can't! You're too weak! You can't take it anymore! You'll never make it! Look how much it hurts! It's not worth it! You're not strong enough! Besides, you are way too fat and it will take forever to lose all of this weight! This is impossible! You can't take this another instant! Eat the donut now! You can always start the diet again tomorrow! You deserve it; you worked hard all week. You have to have SOME fun in life! Forget about the diet and treat yourself! You deserve it! If you turn right on that corner, the donut shop is just a mile down the road! Drive by just to see! Do it now!"

You may relate to this onslaught. Without proper tools, a person that is so assailed will likely find him or herself relapsing.

Sometimes the thoughts are very loud and undeniable. Other times, they can be soft and subtle – almost unconscious. Pause and listen to your mind carefully. You will soon be able to identify the source. If you are not used to listening to your mental chatter, this may initially be a challenge. But I implore you to continue. What we are exploring here holds the keys to your future. It can unlock doors that, up to now, have remained closed in your life.

*Once you have identified the disruptive mental conversation, go back to the serpent. Visualize it twisting and turning upward, attempting to bite you as you hold the tip of its tail with the thumb and forefinger of your right arm.

<u>**THERE**</u> is the thought and/or conversation that is trying to make you fall! <u>**THERE**</u> is the culprit! **You have found the enemy**. You are holding it in your hand. You can now see it. It has been uncovered. Are you now ready to let it go? Do you see that it has been <u>**YOU**</u> holding it all along? Do you

realize that the only power the serpent **EVER** had over you was to convince you to keep holding it, **AND** to continue listening to its lies?

Answer these questions in the silence of your thoughts as you keep your mind's eye fixed on this sleazy, lying serpent squirming and trying to bite you. Let the answers sink deep. **Feel the answers.**

(Example: *"Yes, I see you, you vile filthy serpent! You are the one that has constantly led me to fall. But I have uncovered you, I am aware of your lies, and I am fully ready to release you and vanquish you from my life once and for all."*)

Meanwhile, continue to observe the snake ... do this until you have <u>internalized the dramatic meaning of your discovery</u>. Since you **NOW** can **SEE** the enemy and have become familiar with its **VOICE**, you no longer have to be victimized by it! You are free!

NOW ... visualize yourself *releasing the snake and walking away from it until it is completely gone from sight.* Visualize yourself opening your hand and turning it upward until you can see your palm. Walk away and leave the serpent behind as you see that both of the palms of your hands are empty. You have completely released the serpent and are holding on to nothing.

With each step you take away from the serpent, the negative suggestions, arguments and conversations become dimmer and dimmer.

I like to throw the serpent in pit of fire and hear it screech as it dissolves in the flames. **In the end, the voice is completely gone and you stand in silence and <u>FREEDOM</u>.**

Visualize yourself standing under warm and comfortable sunlight, bright rays hugging your entire being and filling you with power and determination. <u>This is your liberation</u>! You can now walk forward and move directly towards all of your weight loss and health-improvement goals.

Negative Internal Directives

The most common remark I receive at this point is:

"I can release the serpent all day long Robert, but I still feel hungry, dizzy and upset... this RTS business seems like nonsense!"

Yes, you may still feel the hunger and other physical symptoms *(external situation)*, but there will no longer be any <u>negative internal directive</u> *(serpent)* trying to goad you into taking counterproductive actions (*breaking the diet, eating too much, eating between meals, giving in to temptation*).

There is a big difference between: **A)** Experiencing hunger and cravings **WITH** a negative internal voice relentlessly inciting you to give in, and **B)** Experiencing hunger and cravings, but being free of the endless arguments and invitations to break the diet and give up on your goals.

Since the serpent was released and the mental chatter is silenced, the only thing that remains are hunger and cravings.

However, it is much easier to walk through physical discomfort when there is internal silence. External symptoms are fleeting and temporary. By releasing the serpent and refusing to give up, you will find that the hunger and cravings will dissolve in a very short period of time.

The bottom line is this:

Once you release the serpent, you can

handle hunger and cravings as external symptoms <u>WITHOUT</u> breaking your diet. Instead, you can shift your attention to **POSITIVE** actions that can help ease the discomfort as, for example, reading your journal, practicing the *Time Trap Escape* and *Detox Breathing*.

With practice, you will see that these strategies work hand in hand. One builds on top of the other to help you defeat the moment of temptation. The good news is: As you stick to your diet and refuse to give in to temptation, the hunger and cravings will diminish in intensity.

When you least expect it, you will suddenly notice that they have either disappeared altogether or have become just minor irritations. Yes! The symptoms will pass. They always do; and you will be a much leaner and stronger person for having hung on.

<u>Clarification</u>: *Release The Serpent, The Time Trap Escape and Detox Breathing* are by no means exercises that you do **ONCE** and then everything is wonderful for all time. That would be nice, but it unfortunately is not the case.

The mental silence gets longer with practice. At first, however, do these exercises as often as you need to. If you have to go through them ten, twenty, thirty times per day ... so be it. I often find myself constantly releasing the serpent. I get the urge to eat junk food and the mind beckons me to stray. I identify the mental arguments behind the temptation (*"Today is two-for-one peperoni pizzas! Just eat one and work out twice has hard tomorrow" and so on.*) I visualize the snake and identify it as the voice tempting me to stray, I release it and mentally walk away from it. I feel the silence for a few minutes, but then the voice returns and begins to harass me afresh.

So, without delay, I go through the *RTS* exercise again, each time releasing the serpent and looking at my empty palms. I tell myself:

"I have released the serpent and walked away from the constant negative chatter. I feel the silence and my palms are empty; I am holding on to nothing. I can rest without having to give in to this temptation."

Then I swiftly jump into *DB* and/or *The Time Trap Escape.* Sometimes I do this nonstop for days, particularly when I'm feeling vulnerable or am going through a particular trial. I have trained myself to do *RTS*, *DB* and *The Time Trap Escape* automatically. I no longer have to think or force myself to do them. And, after 10+ years, these techniques have never failed me. I can't tell you how many times they have stopped me from giving in to highly-destructive temptations.

Yes, I have saved myself a lot of heartache. Not to mention that I reach my goals much faster because I am not constantly sidetracked by negative mental arguments. Give yourself to the task of practicing these techniques on a daily basis until you fully incorporate them into your thought process. If you do that, it won't be long before you experience a breakthrough.

What is the breakthrough?

Can you imagine yourself capable of facing hunger and cravings and not give in to them? Can you imagine yourself sticking to your diet month after month without further delay or interruptions? Can you imagine the pounds dropping off of your body like never before because you have remained consistent?

How much would all of this be worth to you? The answer is ... **LOTS!** I managed to traverse through horrendous hunger pains and detox symptoms during a 40-day water fast. Apart from the *Grace of God*, these mental techniques were the primary tools that helped me to prevail. Now it is <u>YOUR</u> turn to go all the way and lose every last ounce of excess weight from your body. You can do it; I know that you can!

Assignments

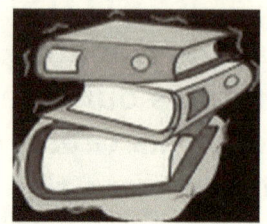

1. **Re-Read this book several times until you fully internalize the techniques that we discussed**.

    Since we are talking about abstract concepts, I want you to take as much time as needed to study and clearly understand the material. This is especially important with the *RTS* concept, which is based on visualization.

    Start immediately to answer the 20 anchor questions outlined in the first part of the book. Remember to purchase a nice journal and not simply write in an old notebook. The journal is going to lead you to deep transformation; so make sure that it is a very special book that you can carry with you at all times. Take your time, but take action.

Never stop reviewing and adding more to each of the answers.

2. **When Hunger, Cravings and the Three Horsemen of Depression, Emotionalism and Impulsivity** (*or other symptoms*) Strike, Immediately **STOP** and read through the journal and, if possible, write a new entry.

Write about how you are feeling at that very moment. (Example: *I feel like crap and just want to eat a pastry because I'm fed up with this diet and can't take it anymore.*)

Carry out the *Time Trap Escape* exercise followed by a ten-minute session of *Detox Breathing*. Do this as many times per day as you have to, ending each session with *Release the Serpent*. Give yourself wholeheartedly to these techniques and do not give up if at first it feels strange and silly.

3. **When you have free moments, feed your mind with DB, The Time Trap Escape and RTS.**

This is basically a way of constantly working out your mental muscles, making them sharp and agile so, when temptation hits, you will be ready. Believe me, when practiced as a lifestyle, these techniques will give you invaluable ammunition to combat and vanquish the thoughts and feelings that will try to knock you off your diet. Stay alert!

4. **Expand the personal journal and spend time daily writing your thoughts and goals**.

As I have said several times, the key to ultimate success in weight loss is your commitment to the process. A life worth living is a life worth recording. The more you write on your journal and log what you are feeling from one moment to another, the harder it will be for temptation to sneak in and knock you off-base.

Most of all, spending time on the journal answering the 20 questions, expanding the answers and writing your personal thoughts will solidity your willingness and desire to change. Why? Because you will be constantly focusing on the strong reasons why it is important for you to lose weight once and for all. Keeping those reasons constantly on your mind is the key to success in weight loss.

You can release the serpent for all eternity, but if you have no real desire to change – then it simply won't work. The desire and willingness to change is what holds everything together. Desire for a better life accompanied by the willingness to walk through the temporary physical discomfort.

* Can you imagine yourself capable of facing hunger and cravings and not give into them?

* Can you imagine yourself sticking to your diet month after month without further delay or interruptions?

* Can you imagine the pounds dropping off of your body like never before because you have remained consistent?

* Can you imagine yourself keeping the weight off year after year and never having to struggle with your weight again?

How much would all of this be worth to you? The answer is ... **LOTS!** And helping you to achieve those goals is exactly what this book is all about. Have you tried to lose weight many times and not succeeded? Have you lost weight in the past but regained it in a matter of months? Do you find yourself *gung-ho* with your diet at one moment, then, just like that, succumb to hunger and or cravings? If so, then you're in the right place.

We all know that sticking to a diet long-term can be a challenge. Wanting to eat in-between meals and struggling with the imperious urge for junk food (*or any other food not in your diet)* are the toughest foes in any weight loss program.

Particularly if you are having a bad day or are otherwise physically or emotionally tired, a sudden assault of hunger and cravings could very well cause one to stray. That is why it is important to have mental tools readily-available that can neutralize these mental enemies before they sabotage your progress.

I was obese and trapped in binge-eating for nearly 25 years, so I know how demoralizing this can be.

The good news is that there is a way out.

Not only did I manage to lose 100 pounds,

but I have kept the weight off for more than 10 years now. In this book, I share with you the mental techniques that helped me walk through temptation and discomfort **WITHOUT** breaking my diet and giving up on my weight loss goals.

Today, these simple but powerful techniques continue to keep my food-related behaviors in check. For the first time in my life, my weight in stable and I'm no longer yo-yoing as I did for so many years. **And what has worked for me and many others can also work for you.**

If you wish to stick to your diet and lose weight once and for all, I invite you to join me in this journey through weight loss and the mind. By practicing and mastering the techniques presented in this book, you'll find inner strength to hang on until the temptation passes. That, in turn, will place you in a direct path with all of your weight loss and health-improvement goals. The time for your breakthrough has arrived!

Finally, Stay Close to <u>AND</u> Communicate frequently with at least one person close to you that you trust and who knows what you are trying to accomplish.

NONE OF US CAN DO THIS ALONE.

I have tried it and, while I made some progress, it eventually did not last. We need each other. So please do not isolate or try to do this alone. And, as I always like to say: When tempted to stray, always remember - Nothing *Tastes as Good as Thin Feels!* God bless and Godspeed.

<u>Grab The Entire Collection!</u>

How to Lose Weight Fast, Keep it Off & Renew the Mind, Body & Spirit through Fasting, Smart Eating & Practical Spirituality

Volume 1: The 'Permanent Weight Loss' Diet

Volume 2: The Intermittent Fasting Weight Loss Formula

Volume 3: How to Lose 30 Pounds (Or More) In 30 Days with Juice Fasting

Volume 4: Burn the Blubber; How to Lose Belly Fat Fast, and For Good!

Volume 5: Lose the Emotional Baggage: Transform Your Mind & Spirit with Fasting

Volume 6: How to Break a Fast and Keep the Weight Off

Volume 7: Compilation Volumes 1-6 -> Get All 6 For The Price Of 4!

Also by Robert Dave Johnston:

How to Lose Weight & Keep it Off by Transforming the Mind & Behaviors

Volume 1: How to Lose Weight & Keep it Off By Reprogramming the Subconscious Mind

Volume 2: Mental Strategies to Defeat Diet Hunger and Junk Food Cravings

Volume 3: The Cravings Ninja Assassin

Volume 4: How to Cheat on Your Diet (And Get Away With It)

Volume 5: Compilation

Detoxify Your Body, Lose Weight, Get Healthy & Transform Your Life

Volume 1: The 10-Day 'At-Home' Colon Cleansing Formula

Volume 2: Bug Off! A 30-Day Parasite, Liver, Kidney Detox & Weight Loss Plan

Volume 3: Lose 30 Pounds (Or More) in 30 Days with Intermittent Fasting & Coffee Enemas

Volume 4: Compilation

Don't forget to check the articles and growing health community at: FitnessThroughFasting.com

Rob's first work of horror/fiction has just been released.
The King of Pain – A Journey to Hell & Back Through the Mind's Eye Volume 1 – The Descent